Dosage Calculations for Nursing Students

Master Dosage Calculations the Safe & Easy Way Without Formulas!

© **Copyright 2024 - All rights reserved.**

The content contained within this book may not be reproduced, duplicated or transmitted without direct written permission from the author or the publisher.

Under no circumstances will any blame or legal responsibility be held against the publisher, or author, for any damages, reparation, or monetary loss due to the information contained within this book. Either directly or indirectly.

Legal Notice:

This book is copyright protected. This book is only for personal use. You cannot amend, distribute, sell, use, quote or paraphrase any part, or the content within this book, without the consent of the author or publisher.

Disclaimer Notice:

Please note the information contained within this document is for educational and entertainment purposes only. All effort has been executed to present accurate, up to date, and reliable, complete information. No warranties of any kind are declared or implied. Readers acknowledge that the author is not engaging in the rendering of legal, financial, medical or professional advice. The content within this book has been derived from various sources. Please consult a licensed professional before attempting any techniques outlined in this book.

By reading this document, the reader agrees that under no circumstances is the author responsible for any losses, direct or indirect, which are incurred as a result of the use of information contained within this document, including, but not limited to, — errors, omissions, or inaccuracies.

DESCRIPTION 4
DESCRIPTION 4
INTRODUCTION 6
CHAPTER 1: UNDERSTANDING DOSAGE CALCULATIONS 8
   1.1 BASICS OF DOSAGE CALCULATIONS 9
   1.2 UNITS OF MEASUREMENT 10
   1.4 READING AND INTERPRETING MEDICATION ORDERS 13
CHAPTER 2: THE FORMULA-FREE APPROACH 16
   2.1 RATIONALE BEHIND THE NO-FORMULA APPROACH 17
   2.2 MASTERING PROPORTIONS THROUGH VISUALIZATION 19
   2.3 ESTIMATION TECHNIQUES 21
   2.4 PRACTICE SCENARIOS 22
CHAPTER 3: APPLICATION IN CLINICAL SETTINGS 24
   3.1 CASE STUDIES 24
   3.2 ERROR PREVENTION 27
   3.3 USING TECHNOLOGY AIDS 29
   3.4 COMMUNICATION AND TEAMWORK 32
CHAPTER 4: SPECIAL CONSIDERATIONS IN DOSAGE CALCULATIONS 35
   4.1 PEDIATRIC DOSAGES 36
   4.2 GERIATRIC DOSAGES 38
   4.3 EMERGENCY SITUATIONS 40
   4.4 HIGH-RISK MEDICATIONS 42
CHAPTER 5: BUILDING CONFIDENCE AND COMPETENCE 45
   5.1 DEVELOPING INTUITION 45
   5.2 CONTINUOUS LEARNING AND IMPROVEMENT 47
   5.3 SIMULATION AND PRACTICE TOOLS 50
   5.4 PREPARING FOR EXAMS 51
CONCLUSION 53

Description

Are you ready to master dosage calculations with ease and confidence, without the burden of complex formulas?

"Dosage Calculations for Nursing Students: Master Dosage Calculations the Safe & Easy Way Without Formulas!" is your essential guide to conquering one of the most crucial skills in nursing. Whether you're a nursing student struggling with traditional methods or a practicing nurse looking to refine your calculation skills, this book offers a fresh, formula-free approach that simplifies the process and boosts your confidence.

This book goes beyond the basics to provide a comprehensive, step-by-step guide to accurate and efficient dosage calculations, all without the need for memorized formulas. You'll learn through intuitive reasoning, practical examples, and real-world scenarios that make complex calculations second nature.

Inside this book, you'll discover:

- **The Formula-Free Approach**: Learn how to perform accurate dosage calculations using intuitive methods, visualization techniques, and proportional reasoning.

- **Real-Life Clinical Scenarios**: Apply what you've learned to real-world nursing situations, including emergency care, pediatric dosing, and high-risk medications.

- **Error Prevention Strategies**: Understand the common pitfalls in dosage calculations and how to avoid them through double-checking, teamwork, and the use of technological aids.

- **Practical Tools and Tips**: Access a variety of simulation tools, practice exercises, and exam preparation strategies that reinforce your skills and build your confidence.

- **Continuous Learning**: Explore resources for ongoing education to ensure your dosage calculation skills remain sharp and up-to-date throughout your nursing career.

Master dosage calculations the safe and easy way, and step into your nursing career with the confidence to deliver exceptional patient care. This book is your pathway to becoming a proficient, confident nurse, ready to tackle any dosage challenge with ease.

Introduction

Imagine a nurse in the hectic environment of an emergency room, where every second counts and every decision has the potential to save a life—or endanger it. In these moments, the ability to calculate a medication dose quickly and accurately is not just a skill; it's a critical component of patient safety. Yet, traditional methods of dosage calculation, often mired in complex formulas and rote memorization, can falter under pressure, leading to hesitation and error. This book, *"Dosage Calculations for Nursing Students: Master Dosage Calculations the Safe & Easy Way Without Formulas!"*, is designed to change that.

Dosage calculations are a cornerstone of nursing practice. Every day, nurses administer medications that must be precisely dosed to ensure their effectiveness and avoid potentially dangerous side effects. Errors in these calculations can lead to underdosing, which may render a treatment ineffective, or overdosing, which can cause serious harm or even be fatal. For nursing students, mastering this skill is not just about passing exams; it's about preparing to deliver safe, competent care in real-world clinical settings.

However, the traditional approach to learning dosage calculations—one that relies heavily on memorizing formulas—presents significant challenges. Many students find these methods frustrating and difficult to retain, especially under the stress of exams or clinical situations. The pressure to remember and correctly apply complex formulas can lead to anxiety and errors, undermining confidence and competence. This book addresses these challenges head-on by offering an alternative: a formula-free approach to dosage calculations that prioritizes understanding and practical application over memorization.

The formula-free approach is an innovative method that simplifies dosage calculations by focusing on intuitive reasoning, visualization, and real-life scenarios. Instead of burdening students with a list of formulas to memorize, this approach encourages a deeper understanding of the principles behind dosage calculations. By using proportional reasoning, estimation techniques, and visual aids, students can learn to perform accurate calculations more naturally and confidently. This method not only enhances accuracy but also speeds up the calculation process, which is crucial in time-sensitive clinical situations. Moreover, it reduces the anxiety associated with traditional methods, making it easier for students to focus on providing excellent patient care.

This book is structured to guide you step by step, from foundational concepts to advanced applications in clinical settings. Each chapter builds on the previous one, gradually enhancing your proficiency and confidence. You'll start with the basics of understanding units of measurement and progress through topics like converting units, reading medication orders, and applying your skills in specialized settings such as pediatrics, geriatrics, and emergency care. Along the way, you'll develop not only the competence to perform dosage calculations but also the confidence to trust your results.

As you embark on this learning journey, remember that the skills you acquire here will serve you well beyond the classroom. They will become an integral part of your nursing practice, enabling you to make quick, accurate decisions that could one day save a life. Embrace the formula-free approach as a powerful tool that will not only help you succeed in your studies but also prepare you for the challenges and rewards of a nursing career dedicated to patient safety and care excellence.

Chapter 1: Understanding Dosage Calculations

Picture yourself in a busy hospital ward, where every second counts. A nurse's responsibility extends far beyond patient care—accuracy in medication dosage is a matter of life and death. Mistakes are not an option. This chapter is your starting point, the foundation upon which all your future clinical skills will be built.

Understanding dosage calculations is not just a technical requirement; it's a core competency that ensures patient safety. Miscalculations can lead to serious consequences, from underdosing to overdosing, both of which can be fatal. The ability to calculate dosages correctly, without relying on complex formulas, is what will set you apart as a competent, confident nurse.

In this chapter, we will explore the basics of dosage calculations, delve into the different units of measurement, and guide you through the process of converting those units with ease. You'll also learn how to read and interpret medication orders accurately, a skill that will be indispensable throughout your nursing career.

This isn't just about numbers; it's about making sure every patient receives the correct amount of medication, ensuring their safety and recovery. By the end of this chapter, you'll have a solid grasp of the essential skills needed to master dosage calculations and prevent errors in your practice.

1.1 Basics of Dosage Calculations

Dosage calculations are a critical aspect of nursing practice, rooted in the very fabric of medical history. From the earliest apothecaries to modern healthcare systems, the precise measurement of medication has been a cornerstone of effective treatment. The practice of dosage calculation dates back to ancient times when healers relied on rudimentary methods to prepare medicines. Over centuries, as medical science evolved, so did the methods for calculating dosages, leading to the standardized systems we use today.

In nursing, dosage calculations involve determining the correct amount of medication to administer to a patient based on several factors, including the prescribed dose, the patient's weight or age, and the concentration of the medication available. It's a process that demands both accuracy and attention to detail, as even the smallest error can have significant consequences. For example, calculating the wrong dose could lead to an underdose, where the patient doesn't receive enough medication to be effective, or an overdose, which can result in serious harm or even death.

At its core, a dosage calculation in nursing is the process of translating a physician's prescription into the exact amount of medication a patient should receive. This often requires converting units of measurement, adjusting for patient-specific factors like age or body mass, and ensuring that the final calculation is precise. The nurse must then administer this calculated dose accurately, often under time pressure and in high-stress environments.

The importance of accuracy in dosage calculations cannot be overstated. Medication errors are a leading cause of adverse effects in healthcare settings, and many of these errors stem from incorrect dosage calculations. In a profession where precision is paramount, the ability to calculate and administer the correct dose of medication is not just a technical skill—it's a moral obligation. Every dosage you calculate has the potential to affect a patient's recovery, quality of life, and, in some cases, their survival.

Moreover, precision in dosage calculations is a direct reflection of a nurse's competence. It builds trust between the nurse and the patient, as well as among the healthcare team. When a nurse consistently administers the correct dosage, it reinforces the safety and efficacy of the treatment plan. Conversely, errors can lead to a loss of confidence and may result in legal implications for the nurse and the healthcare facility.

In summary, dosage calculations are an integral part of nursing that combines mathematical precision with clinical judgment. Understanding the basics of these calculations is essential for ensuring patient safety and providing high-quality care. As you progress in your nursing career, mastering this skill will become second nature, but it starts with a solid understanding of the fundamental concepts. In the next sections, we'll build on this foundation, exploring the units of measurement and the techniques used to ensure accuracy in every dosage calculation you perform.

1.2 Units of Measurement

In the world of medication dosage, understanding units of measurement is essential. Accurate dosing depends on the nurse's ability to interpret and convert between different measurement systems. This section will guide you through the three main systems you'll encounter: the metric system, the apothecary system, and the household measurement system.

The Metric System

The metric system is the most commonly used measurement system in healthcare today, favored for its simplicity and precision. It is based on units of ten, making conversions straightforward and less prone to error. The primary units of measurement in the metric system that you'll encounter include:

- **Gram (g)**: Used for measuring mass. In dosage calculations, you'll often see this in milligrams (mg) or micrograms (mcg), which are smaller units.

- **Liter (L)**: Used for measuring volume. Milliliters (mL) are commonly used in dosing, especially for liquid medications.

- **Meter (m)**: Though less common in dosage calculations, meters may be used in measuring body height, which can be relevant in calculating doses based on body surface area.

For example, a typical prescription might call for 500 mg of a medication, which is a straightforward application of the metric system. Understanding how to move between grams, milligrams, and micrograms is crucial. Remember, 1 gram equals 1,000 milligrams, and 1 milligram equals 1,000 micrograms.

Converting Pounds to Kilograms: Since many caregivers may provide a child's weight in pounds (lb), it's essential to know how to convert this to kilograms, as most pediatric dosages are calculated in metric units. The conversion is straightforward:

$$\text{Weight (kg)} = \frac{\text{Weight (lb)}}{2.2}$$

For example, if a child weighs 44 lb, converting this to kilograms would involve dividing 44 by 2.2, resulting in a weight of 20 kg.

The Apothecary System

The apothecary system is older and less frequently used in modern medicine, but it's still important to be familiar with it, especially when dealing with certain medications. The apothecary system uses different units:

- **Grain (gr)**: A unit of weight commonly seen in older prescriptions or specific medications, particularly for thyroid hormones or aspirin.

- **Minim (min)** and **dram (dr)**: Units of volume that are less frequently encountered but are still relevant in some cases.

For instance, a prescription might state that a patient needs 5 grains of a medication. Knowing that 1 grain is approximately 64.8 milligrams is essential for converting this to a more familiar metric unit.

The Household Measurement System

The household measurement system is used more in patient education, particularly for over-the-counter medications or home care. It includes units like:

- **Teaspoon (tsp)**: Equivalent to 5 mL.
- **Tablespoon (tbsp)**: Equivalent to 15 mL.
- **Ounce (oz)**: Typically, 1 fluid ounce equals 30 mL.

These units are often used when explaining dosages to patients, particularly in home settings where medications might be measured using kitchen utensils. For example, a dose might be 2 teaspoons of a liquid medication, which the nurse knows equates to 10 mL.

Tips for Remembering and Converting Units

Converting between these units can be challenging, but with a few tips, it becomes more manageable:

- **Mnemonic devices**: Create simple phrases to remember conversions, such as "King Henry Died By Drinking Chocolate Milk" to recall kilo, hecto, deka, base, deci, centi, milli.
- **Flashcards**: Use flashcards to drill conversions, especially between metric units.
- **Practice problems**: The more you practice, the more intuitive these conversions will become.

For instance, to convert 2 grams to milligrams, you simply multiply by 1,000, resulting in 2,000 mg. This straightforward approach is what makes the metric system so valuable in clinical settings.

In conclusion, understanding the various units of measurement and how to convert between them is a foundational skill in nursing. Whether you're dealing with metric, apothecary, or household units, accuracy in these conversions is essential for safe and effective patient care. As we move forward, we'll apply these units to real-world dosage calculations, ensuring that you are well-prepared for clinical practice.

1.4 Reading and Interpreting Medication Orders

Reading and interpreting medication orders is a crucial skill that every nurse must master to ensure patient safety and effective treatment. Medication orders are instructions provided by a physician or authorized prescriber detailing the specific drug, dosage, route of administration, and timing for a patient. Misinterpreting these orders can lead to medication errors, which can have serious consequences. In this section, we'll break down the key components of medication orders, discuss common abbreviations and medical terminology, and provide strategies for clarifying and verifying orders when needed.

Understanding Common Abbreviations and Medical Terminology

Medication orders often include a variety of abbreviations and medical terms that can be confusing, especially for those new to nursing. Familiarity with these abbreviations is essential for accurate interpretation. Here are some of the most common ones you'll encounter:

- q.d. (quaque die): **Once a day**
- b.i.d. (bis in die): **Twice a day**
- t.i.d. (ter in die): Three times a day
- q.i.d. (quater in die): **Four times a day**
- PRN (pro re nata): **As needed**
- PO (per os): **By mouth**

- **IV (intravenous)**: Administered through a vein
- **IM (intramuscular)**: Administered into a muscle
- **mg (milligrams)**: A unit of mass for the medication dose
- **mL (milliliters)**: A unit of volume for liquid medications

For example, an order reading "Aspirin 325 mg PO q.d." means the patient should receive 325 milligrams of aspirin by mouth once a day. Understanding these abbreviations ensures that you administer the medication correctly according to the physician's instructions.

How to Clarify and Verify Unclear Orders

Despite the best efforts of prescribers, sometimes medication orders can be unclear or ambiguous. When faced with an order that is difficult to interpret, it's essential to take the necessary steps to clarify the information before administering any medication. Here's how to handle such situations:

1. **Double-check the order**: Compare the order with the patient's chart, previous prescriptions, and the standard dosage for the medication. This might provide context or clarification.

2. **Consult with colleagues**: Ask a fellow nurse or a pharmacist if they can help clarify the order. Sometimes, another set of eyes can catch something you might have missed.

3. **Contact the prescriber**: If there is still any doubt, reach out to the prescribing physician for clarification. It's better to ask and be certain than to guess and potentially harm the patient.

For instance, if an order reads "Lasix 40 mg IV q.d.," but the patient's chart suggests they normally receive it b.i.d., it's critical to verify with the prescriber before proceeding.

Examples of Medication Orders and How to Interpret Them

Let's look at a few examples of medication orders and how to interpret them correctly:

1. **Order**: "Tylenol 500 mg PO q6h PRN for pain."

    - **Interpretation**: Administer 500 milligrams of Tylenol by mouth every six hours as needed for pain relief.

    - **Order**: "Heparin 5,000 units subQ b.i.d."

    - **Interpretation**: Administer 5,000 units of Heparin subcutaneously (under the skin) twice a day.

    - **Order**: "Vancomycin 1 g IV over 60 min q12h."

    - **Interpretation**: Administer 1 gram of Vancomycin intravenously over 60 minutes every 12 hours.

These examples illustrate the importance of accurately interpreting each part of the order—drug, dose, route, and timing—to ensure the medication is administered safely and effectively.

Accurately reading and interpreting medication orders is a vital skill for nurses, directly impacting patient safety and treatment outcomes. By understanding common abbreviations and medical terminology, and knowing when and how to clarify unclear orders, you can confidently prepare and administer medications as prescribed. This attention to detail not only ensures compliance with the physician's instructions but also safeguards the well-being of your patients. As you continue to build your nursing skills, this proficiency will become an invaluable part of your daily practice.

Chapter 2: The Formula-Free Approach

Imagine walking into a room with complete confidence, ready to calculate the exact dosage a patient needs without hesitation. This confidence stems from a method that strips away the complexity of traditional formulas and replaces it with a more intuitive approach—one that aligns with how our minds naturally work. Welcome to the formula-free approach to dosage calculations.

Traditional methods often overwhelm nursing students with endless formulas and equations, leading to confusion and mistakes. The formula-free approach challenges this by simplifying the process, making it more accessible and less intimidating. Instead of memorizing abstract formulas, you'll learn to rely on visualization, estimation, and proportion—a method that not only simplifies calculations but also enhances your understanding and retention of key concepts.

This chapter will introduce you to the core philosophy behind this approach, showing how it fits seamlessly into modern nursing practices. You'll discover how this method improves real-world application, allowing you to perform calculations quickly and accurately, even under pressure. The goal is simple: to empower you with a practical, reliable method that you can trust in any clinical setting.

By the end of this chapter, you'll understand why the formula-free approach is more than just an alternative—it's a powerful tool that can transform your practice and boost your confidence as a nurse.

2.1 Rationale Behind the No-Formula Approach

The no-formula approach to dosage calculations is grounded in a deep understanding of how our brains process and retain information. Cognitive load theory, a principle widely recognized in educational psychology, suggests that our working memory has a limited capacity. When this capacity is overloaded—such as when trying to remember and apply complex formulas—our ability to process information and make accurate decisions diminishes. The no-formula approach seeks to reduce this cognitive load by removing the need for rote memorization of formulas, allowing you to focus on understanding and applying concepts more intuitively.

Traditional methods of dosage calculation often require students to memorize a variety of formulas, each tailored to specific types of calculations. For instance, you might be expected to remember formulas for calculating dosages based on weight, adjusting doses for pediatric patients, or converting units between different measurement systems. While these formulas can be effective, they also impose a significant cognitive burden. Each new formula adds to the load on your working memory, increasing the chances of errors, particularly in high-pressure situations where quick decisions are required.

The no-formula approach, on the other hand, simplifies the process by encouraging the use of proportional reasoning and estimation—techniques that align more closely with natural cognitive processes. For example, rather than relying on a specific formula to calculate a dose, you might use visual aids or simple ratios that can be easily recalled and applied in various contexts. This reduces the cognitive strain and allows you to perform calculations more efficiently and with greater confidence.

Consider a common scenario in nursing practice: calculating the correct dose of a medication based on a patient's weight. The traditional method might involve a specific formula where you input the patient's weight, the prescribed dose, and the concentration of the drug to arrive at the correct dosage. This process requires you to remember and correctly apply the formula, which can be challenging, especially under stress.

In contrast, the no-formula approach would have you use proportional reasoning. You might start by determining the dose for a standard weight (e.g., per kilogram) and then simply multiply by the patient's weight. This method is not only easier to understand but also more adaptable across different scenarios, reducing the likelihood of errors.

Research supports the effectiveness of intuitive learning methods like the no-formula approach. Studies have shown that when learners engage with material in a way that reduces cognitive load, they are better able to retain and apply that information in practical settings. For example, a study published in the *Journal of Nursing Education* found that students who were taught using visual aids and proportional reasoning techniques performed better on dosage calculation tests than those who relied on traditional formula-based methods. These students also reported higher levels of confidence in their ability to perform dosage calculations in clinical practice.

Moreover, the no-formula approach aligns with the principles of experiential learning, where knowledge is constructed through real-life experiences rather than abstract concepts. Nurses who learn through intuitive methods are more likely to retain their skills and apply them effectively in diverse clinical situations. This approach not only enhances immediate performance but also contributes to long-term competency in nursing practice.

In summary, the no-formula approach offers a more effective and efficient way to master dosage calculations. By reducing cognitive load and focusing on intuitive learning methods, this approach helps you process information more effectively, retain critical skills, and apply them confidently in the clinical setting. It's a method designed to enhance your understanding, improve accuracy, and ultimately, provide safer patient care.

2.2 Mastering Proportions through Visualization

Proportional reasoning is at the heart of dosage calculations and mastering this skill can be significantly enhanced through visualization techniques. By transforming abstract numbers into concrete images, you can simplify complex calculations and improve both your understanding and accuracy. Visualization not only makes the math more intuitive but also reduces the cognitive load, allowing you to focus on the practical application of your knowledge.

Visual Tools: Diagrams and Proportional Circles

One of the most effective visual tools for mastering proportions is the proportional circle, a simple yet powerful diagram that helps you visualize ratios and relationships between different quantities. Imagine you need to calculate a medication dosage based on a specific patient weight. Instead of relying on a formula, you can use a proportional circle to map out the relationship between the standard dose and the patient's weight, making the calculation process more intuitive.

For instance, let's say a standard dose of a medication is 10 mg for a patient weighing 50 kg. To find the correct dose for a patient weighing 70 kg, draw a circle and divide it into segments representing the doses and corresponding weights. The visualization clearly shows the proportional relationship, making it easier to calculate the dosage without memorizing a formula. In this case, if 10 mg corresponds to 50 kg, then 14 mg would correspond to 70 kg—a straightforward calculation made even clearer through visual representation.

Step-by-Step Example Using Proportional Circles

Let's walk through a specific example to illustrate how proportional circles can be applied to dosage calculations:

Scenario: You need to calculate the dosage of a medication that is prescribed at 5 mg per 20 kg of body weight. The patient weighs 60 kg.

1. **Draw the Proportional Circle**: Start by drawing a circle. Inside the circle, write down the known values: 5 mg in one segment and 20 kg in the corresponding segment.

2. **Determine the Unknown Quantity**: You know the patient's weight is 60 kg, so you need to calculate the corresponding dose. Since 60 kg is three times 20 kg, you can visually represent this by extending the segments in the circle—if 5 mg corresponds to 20 kg, then the dose for 60 kg would be three times 5 mg, or 15 mg.

3. **Visual Confirmation**: The proportional circle allows you to see at a glance that the ratio is maintained, reinforcing the accuracy of your calculation.

This method not only simplifies the process but also helps prevent common errors that can occur when relying solely on numerical formulas. The visual aid serves as a quick check to ensure that the ratios align correctly, making the process both faster and more reliable.

The Importance of Visual Learning Aids

Visual aids like proportional circles are more than just tools for simplifying calculations—they are essential for enhancing comprehension and retention. Studies in educational psychology have shown that visual learning significantly improves understanding and recall, especially when dealing with complex concepts like dosage calculations. When you see the relationships between quantities laid out visually, the information is more likely to be stored in long-term memory, reducing the need for repetitive memorization.

Moreover, visual aids help bridge the gap between theory and practice. In a clinical setting, where quick and accurate decisions are critical, being able to visualize the proportional relationships in dosage calculations can lead to faster, more confident decision-making. This is particularly important under pressure, where traditional formulas might lead to hesitation or error.

Mastering proportions through visualization is a powerful strategy for dosage calculations. By using tools like proportional circles, you can make complex calculations more intuitive and less error-prone. This approach not only enhances your ability to perform accurate calculations but also builds your confidence in real-world clinical situations. As you continue to develop your skills, these visual techniques will become an invaluable part of your nursing practice, helping you to deliver safe and effective patient care.

2.3 Estimation Techniques

Estimation is a valuable skill in nursing, especially when time is of the essence. In clinical settings, the ability to quickly and accurately estimate dosages can make a significant difference in patient outcomes. Estimation techniques, when combined with the no-formula approach, provide a practical and efficient way to handle dosage calculations without getting bogged down in complex math.

Understanding Benchmark Dosages

A benchmark dosage is a standard or reference point that you can use to estimate other doses. It's a known quantity that serves as a baseline, allowing you to make quick, proportional adjustments based on patient-specific factors. For instance, if you know that 10 mg of a certain medication is the appropriate dose for a 50 kg patient, this can serve as your benchmark. From this point, you can easily estimate the dose for patients of different weights without needing to calculate it precisely each time.

Example: If 10 mg is the dose for 50 kg, then for a patient weighing 100 kg, you can quickly estimate the dose to be 20 mg—simply doubling the benchmark dose since the patient's weight is doubled. This estimation technique leverages proportional reasoning, making it faster and easier than traditional calculation methods.

Applying Estimation in Real Scenarios

Let's look at a practical example where estimation can be used effectively:

Scenario: You are administering a drug that is typically dosed at 0.5 mg per kg of body weight. Your patient weighs 75 kg. Instead of reaching for a calculator, you can use estimation.

1. **Identify the Benchmark**: Let's use 1 mg for a 2 kg patient as a simple benchmark.

2. **Estimate Based on Benchmark**: Since the patient weighs 75 kg, you can estimate the dosage by scaling the benchmark. If 1 mg corresponds to 2 kg, then 75 kg would correspond to 37.5 mg (as 75 is approximately 37.5 times 2). This quick estimation gives you a reliable dosage without the need for precise calculation.

Another approach is to round numbers to make mental calculations easier. For instance, if the weight is slightly above or below a round number (e.g., 74 kg instead of 75 kg), you can round to the nearest simple figure to make the estimation process even quicker.

Enhancing Speed and Confidence

Estimation is not just about speed; it's also about confidence. In high-pressure situations, nurses need to trust their judgment and make decisions quickly. Estimation techniques allow you to bypass the time-consuming steps of formulaic calculations, giving you the confidence to administer doses accurately and efficiently. This is especially crucial when dealing with emergency situations where every second counts.

Moreover, estimation helps build mental agility. As you practice these techniques, you'll find that your ability to estimate dosages accurately improves, reducing the likelihood of errors and enhancing your overall effectiveness in patient care.

2.4 Practice Scenarios

To solidify your understanding of the formula-free approach, it's important to apply these techniques in realistic scenarios. Below are a few practice situations designed to help you reinforce your skills in visualization and estimation.

Scenario 1: Calculating Liquid Medication Dosage

- **Patient Information**: The prescription is for a 60 kg adult patient who needs 15 mg of a liquid medication that is supplied as 5 mg per mL.

- **Task**: Estimate how many milliliters you should administer.

- **Solution**: Using the proportional circle technique, if 5 mg corresponds to 1 mL, then 15 mg would correspond to 3 mL. Thus, the correct dosage is 3 mL.

Scenario 2: Estimating Pediatric Dosage

- **Patient Information**: A child weighs 20 kg, and the medication is typically dosed at 0.25 mg/kg.

- **Task**: Estimate the total dosage.

- **Solution**: Benchmarking at 0.25 mg for each kg, for a 20 kg child, you can estimate the dose to be 5 mg (since 20 times 0.25 equals 5).

Scenario 3: Emergency Estimation for Adult Patient

- **Patient Information**: An adult patient requires an immediate dose of a drug that is generally administered at 1 mg per 10 kg of body weight. The patient weighs 85 kg.

- **Task**: Estimate the dose quickly.

- **Solution**: Rounding the weight to 90 kg for simplicity, estimate the dosage at 9 mg, providing a quick and safe dose in a time-critical situation.

Practice with these scenarios to build confidence and proficiency in using the formula-free approach. The more you apply these techniques, the more intuitive and reliable they will become, making you better prepared to handle dosage calculations in any clinical situation.

Chapter 3: Application in Clinical Settings

Stepping onto the clinical floor for the first time can be both exciting and intimidating. As a nurse, every decision you make has a direct impact on patient care, and accurate dosage calculation is one of the most critical skills you'll use. The formula-free approach you've learned so far is more than just a method—it's a practical tool designed to enhance your confidence and effectiveness in real-world scenarios.

In clinical practice, the ability to apply dosage calculations quickly and accurately is vital. Whether you're in a high-pressure emergency room or a quiet pediatric ward, the decisions you make must be precise and informed by both theoretical knowledge and practical experience. This chapter focuses on how to seamlessly integrate what you've learned about dosage calculations into the fast-paced, often unpredictable environment of clinical care.

We'll explore real-life case studies that demonstrate the effectiveness of the formula-free approach in diverse settings, from critical care to long-term management. You'll learn about common errors and how to prevent them, the role of technology in supporting your calculations, and the importance of communication and teamwork in ensuring patient safety. As you read through this chapter, think about how these strategies can be applied in your own practice, making every calculation a confident step toward better patient outcomes.

3.1 Case Studies

Understanding how to apply dosage calculations in real-world settings is crucial for any nursing student. The following case studies illustrate how the formula-free approach can be successfully implemented in various clinical scenarios. Each example highlights the decision-making process, the outcomes, and key reflections that offer valuable insights for your practice.

Case Study 1: Emergency Care - Rapid Dosage Adjustment

Scenario: A 65-year-old male patient arrives at the emergency department with acute pulmonary edema. The attending physician orders an immediate intravenous (IV) dose of furosemide, a potent diuretic, to reduce fluid overload. The standard dose is 0.5 mg per kilogram of body weight. The patient weighs 80 kg.

Application: In the urgency of the situation, there's no time to rely on a calculator or formulas. Using the formula-free approach, the nurse quickly estimates the required dose. Knowing that 0.5 mg per kg for an 80 kg patient would be approximately 40 mg, the nurse prepares and administers the dose without hesitation.

Outcome: The patient's condition stabilizes as the diuretic begins to take effect. The rapid yet accurate dosage calculation prevented a potentially life-threatening delay, showcasing the effectiveness of the formula-free approach in emergency situations.

Reflection: This case underscores the importance of speed and accuracy in emergency care. The formula-free method allows nurses to make quick, reliable decisions when time is critical, reducing the risk of error and improving patient outcomes.

Case Study 2: Pediatric Care - Weight-Based Dosing

Scenario: A 4-year-old child weighing 20 kg is admitted for treatment of a severe bacterial infection. The physician prescribes an antibiotic that requires a dosage of 25 mg per kilogram, administered intravenously every 8 hours.

Application: The nurse uses proportional reasoning to calculate the correct dose. With the formula-free approach, the nurse quickly estimates that 25 mg per kg for a 20 kg child results in a 500 mg dose. The medication is prepared and administered according to the estimated calculation.

Outcome: The child's infection begins to respond to the antibiotic therapy without any adverse effects from incorrect dosing. The nurse's quick and accurate calculation ensures that the child receives the appropriate care without delay.

Reflection: Pediatric dosing requires careful consideration due to the variability in weight and the sensitivity of young patients to medications. The formula-free approach simplifies the process, allowing nurses to confidently calculate and administer the correct doses, even under pressure.

Case Study 3: Geriatric Care - Dose Adjustment for Renal Impairment

Scenario: An 82-year-old female patient with chronic kidney disease is prescribed digoxin, a medication used to treat heart conditions. The patient's renal function is compromised, requiring a reduced dosage to prevent toxicity. The standard dose is 0.125 mg, but the doctor suggests reducing it by 25%.

Application: Instead of applying a formula, the nurse uses the formula-free approach to adjust the dose. Knowing that 25% of 0.125 mg is approximately 0.03 mg, the nurse subtracts this from the standard dose, arriving at a new dose of approximately 0.09 mg. The nurse rounds this to the nearest safe administration dose, ensuring accuracy.

Outcome: The adjusted dose is administered safely, and the patient's heart condition is managed without signs of digoxin toxicity. The nurse's ability to accurately adjust the dosage based on the patient's renal function highlights the flexibility of the formula-free approach in complex situations.

Reflection: Geriatric patients often require tailored dosages due to comorbidities and organ function decline. The formula-free method allows nurses to make precise adjustments based on individual patient needs, ensuring both efficacy and safety in medication administration.

Key Takeaways

These case studies demonstrate the versatility and effectiveness of the formula-free approach across different clinical settings. Whether in the high-stakes environment of emergency care, the precise demands of pediatric dosing, or the careful adjustments required in geriatric care, this method provides a reliable, intuitive way to ensure accurate medication administration. As you encounter similar scenarios in your practice, remember these examples and the confidence that comes with mastering this approach.

3.2 Error Prevention

Dosage calculation errors can have serious consequences, ranging from ineffective treatment to life-threatening complications. Preventing these errors is critical in nursing practice, and the formula-free approach can play a significant role in reducing mistakes. This section will explore common dosage calculation errors, their potential impacts, and strategies for preventing them using practical methods.

Common Dosage Calculation Errors and Their Consequences

1. Incorrect Unit Conversions: Miscalculations often occur when converting between different units, such as milligrams to grams or milliliters to liters. A small mistake in conversion can lead to a significant error in dosage, potentially resulting in underdosing or overdosing. For example, confusing milligrams (mg) with micrograms (mcg) could lead to administering 1,000 times more medication than intended.

2. Misinterpreting Medication Orders: Errors can also arise from misunderstanding the physician's instructions. This includes misreading abbreviations, confusing similar-sounding medications, or overlooking important details in the order, such as the correct frequency or route of administration. Such errors can lead to administering the wrong dose, at the wrong time, or even the wrong medication.

3. Calculation Errors Due to Complex Formulas: Traditional formula-based methods can be prone to mistakes, especially under pressure. The complexity of some formulas may lead to incorrect application or misinterpretation, resulting in inaccurate dosages.

Strategies for Error Prevention

1. Double-Checking Techniques: One of the simplest yet most effective strategies for preventing errors is double-checking your work. After calculating a dosage using the formula-free approach, verify the result by cross-referencing it with standard dosage charts or guidelines. This step helps catch any potential mistakes before the medication is administered.

2. Peer Reviews: Collaborating with colleagues can further reduce the risk of errors. Before administering a high-risk medication or an unusually large or small dose, ask a peer to review your calculations. A second set of eyes can identify errors you might have missed and provide additional reassurance that the dose is correct.

3. Use of Technological Aids: While the formula-free approach emphasizes manual calculation techniques, technology can still play a supportive role. Digital calculators, apps, and software designed for dosage calculations can serve as tools to verify your estimates. These aids can be particularly useful in complex scenarios where manual calculations might be prone to error. However, it's essential to maintain a strong understanding of the underlying principles so that you can catch any anomalies or inaccuracies in the technology's output.

Importance of Attention to Detail and Thorough Patient Assessment

Attention to detail is paramount in dosage calculations. Small oversights, such as failing to account for a patient's renal function or not considering drug interactions, can lead to significant errors. A thorough patient assessment, including a review of their medical history, current medications, and any relevant lab results, is crucial in ensuring that the dosage is appropriate for their specific situation.

For example, a patient with impaired kidney function may require a reduced dosage of a medication that is primarily excreted by the kidneys. Without this adjustment, the patient could be at risk of toxicity. By carefully assessing the patient's overall condition and considering all relevant factors, you can make informed decisions that enhance patient safety.

In addition, always consider the patient's weight, age, and any allergies or sensitivities when calculating dosages. These factors are integral to determining the correct dose and ensuring that the treatment is both safe and effective.

Key Takeaways

Preventing dosage calculation errors is a critical aspect of nursing practice. The formula-free approach, combined with double-checking techniques, peer reviews, and the judicious use of technology, provides a robust framework for minimizing mistakes. Attention to detail and thorough patient assessment are also essential components of error prevention. By integrating these strategies into your practice, you can significantly reduce the risk of dosage errors, ensuring better patient outcomes and safer care.

3.3 Using Technology Aids

In the fast-paced environment of healthcare, technology aids can significantly enhance the accuracy and efficiency of dosage calculations. While the formula-free approach emphasizes manual calculation techniques, integrating technology can provide an additional layer of safety and convenience. This section will review various technology aids that support nursing dosage calculations, offer examples of their effective use, and discuss the importance of balancing technology reliance with manual skills.

Types of Technology Aids

1. Digital Calculators: Digital calculators are basic yet essential tools in nursing. They allow for quick arithmetic operations and conversions, making it easier to double-check manual calculations. Many calculators designed specifically for healthcare professionals include functions for common dosage calculations, such as drug dilutions and unit conversions.

2. Mobile Apps: Numerous mobile apps are available to assist with dosage calculations. These apps often include features like dosage calculators, drug databases, and unit converters. Some popular apps even offer built-in safety checks that alert users to potential dosing errors based on the patient's weight, age, or renal function. Examples include Medscape, Epocrates, and Calculate by QxMD.

3. Clinical Software: Many hospitals and clinics use integrated clinical software that includes dosage calculation tools as part of the electronic health record (EHR) system. These tools automatically pull patient data, such as weight and age, to calculate dosages, minimizing the risk of human error. Additionally, some systems are linked to pharmacy databases, providing real-time updates on drug interactions and contraindications.

Effective Use of Technology Aids

While technology aids can streamline the dosage calculation process, it's crucial to use them effectively. Here are some guidelines:

1. Verify Manual Calculations: Use technology as a secondary check rather than the primary method. For instance, after performing a manual calculation using the formula-free approach, input the same values into a digital calculator or app to confirm the result. This dual-layered approach helps catch any errors that might have occurred in the manual process.

2. Understand the Principles: Even when using technology, understanding the underlying principles of dosage calculations is essential. Relying solely on technology without comprehension can lead to complacency and increase the risk of errors if the technology malfunctions or provides incorrect data. For example, if an app suggests a dosage that seems unusually high or low, your knowledge of standard dosing should prompt you to investigate further before administering the medication.

3. Regularly Update Tools: Ensure that the apps and software you use are up-to-date with the latest clinical guidelines and drug information. Regular updates are necessary to maintain accuracy, particularly with the frequent changes in drug dosages, formulations, and contraindications.

Balancing Technology and Manual Skills

While technology can enhance the accuracy and efficiency of dosage calculations, it's important not to become overly reliant on it. Manual calculation skills are critical for situations where technology may not be available, such as during power outages or when technology fails. Moreover, manual calculations help reinforce your understanding of dosage principles, making you a more competent and confident nurse.

For example, in a scenario where the EHR system is down, your ability to quickly calculate dosages manually ensures that patient care continues without interruption. Additionally, manual skills are essential for interpreting and verifying the outputs provided by technological tools, ensuring that the calculations make sense in the context of the patient's overall treatment plan.

Key Takeaways

Technology aids, such as digital calculators, mobile apps, and clinical software, can be valuable tools in supporting the formula-free approach to dosage calculations. They provide quick verification, reduce the risk of errors, and offer real-time data integration. However, maintaining a strong foundation in manual calculation skills is equally important. By balancing technology with a solid understanding of dosage principles, you can ensure safe, accurate, and effective patient care, even in challenging situations.

3.4 Communication and Teamwork

Accurate dosage calculations are not just a solitary task—they often require collaboration and clear communication within the healthcare team. Effective communication ensures that every member of the team is on the same page, reducing the risk of errors and enhancing patient safety. This section will explore the importance of communication and teamwork in dosage calculations, provide real-life examples, and offer practical tips for improving communication in clinical settings.

The Importance of Communication in Dosage Calculations

Communication with other healthcare professionals is crucial in the preparation and administration of medications. Misunderstandings or miscommunications can lead to dosage errors, which can have serious consequences for patients. For instance, a physician might prescribe a medication with specific instructions for dosing, and it is the nurse's responsibility to clarify any ambiguities before administration. This might involve confirming the patient's weight, understanding the precise timing of doses, or discussing potential interactions with other medications the patient is taking.

Clear communication is particularly important in situations where multiple team members are involved in the medication process. For example, a pharmacist might prepare the medication, while the nurse administers it, and the physician monitors the patient's response. Any breakdown in communication at these stages can result in errors, making it essential for all parties to share accurate information and confirm understanding.

Teamwork in Solving Complex Dosage Calculations

Teamwork often plays a key role in solving complex dosage calculations, especially in high-pressure environments like emergency rooms or intensive care units. In these settings, nurses, pharmacists, and physicians frequently collaborate to ensure that dosages are calculated correctly and administered safely. For example, in cases involving weight-based dosing for critically ill patients, the team may need to quickly adjust dosages based on fluctuating patient conditions. Working together, they can cross-check calculations, share insights, and ensure that the final dosage is safe and effective.

One scenario might involve a nurse who identifies a potential discrepancy in a medication order. Instead of making a unilateral decision, the nurse brings the issue to the attention of the pharmacist and physician. Through discussion and collaboration, the team can reassess the patient's needs, adjust the dosage if necessary, and ensure that the correct amount is administered. This collaborative approach not only prevents errors but also fosters a culture of safety and shared responsibility.

Tips for Improving Communication in Healthcare Teams

1. **Clarify and Confirm**: Always clarify any unclear instructions or orders with the prescribing physician or pharmacist. Confirm the details before proceeding with dosage calculations or administration.

2. **Use Closed-Loop Communication**: Repeat back the information shared to confirm accuracy. For example, when receiving a verbal order, say, "You're prescribing 50 mg of Drug X to be administered intravenously over 30 minutes, correct?"

3. **Regular Briefings and Debriefings**: In fast-paced environments, regular team briefings and debriefings help ensure everyone is aware of patient status, medication orders, and any recent changes. This reduces the risk of miscommunication.

4. **Foster a Supportive Environment**: Encourage team members to speak up if they notice a potential issue or have a concern. A culture where everyone feels comfortable raising questions is key to preventing errors.

Key Takeaways

Effective communication and teamwork are essential components of accurate dosage calculations. By ensuring clear communication and fostering collaboration within healthcare teams, you can significantly reduce the risk of errors and enhance patient safety. Regularly practicing these communication strategies will help you become a more effective and reliable member of the healthcare team, particularly in high-pressure or complex situations.

Chapter 4: Special Considerations in Dosage Calculations

Accurate dosage calculations are never a one-size-fits-all process. Different patient populations, such as children, the elderly, and those in critical conditions, present unique challenges that require careful consideration. Tailoring dosages to meet the specific needs of these groups is essential to ensure safety and efficacy in treatment.

Children, for example, metabolize medications differently than adults, necessitating precise adjustments based on weight and developmental stage. In contrast, elderly patients often face issues related to slowed metabolism and multiple medications, increasing the risk of interactions and side effects. Emergency situations add another layer of complexity, where decisions must be made quickly, often under immense pressure.

This chapter will explore the critical factors that influence dosage calculations across these varied scenarios. Understanding the variability in patient responses to medications is crucial in nursing, as it ensures that each patient receives the most appropriate care. Through practical examples and actionable strategies, you'll gain the insights needed to navigate these special considerations with confidence and precision, ultimately enhancing patient safety and treatment outcomes.

4.1 Pediatric Dosages

Calculating dosages for pediatric patients requires a different approach than for adults. Children are not simply "small adults"; their bodies process medications in unique ways, which means dosages must be carefully tailored to avoid underdosing or overdosing. The primary factors in pediatric dosage calculations are body weight and surface area, which serve as the foundation for determining the correct dose.

Importance of Body Weight and Surface Area

Pediatric dosages are typically calculated based on the child's weight (in kilograms) or, in some cases, their body surface area (BSA). Weight-based dosing ensures that the medication is proportional to the child's size, which is critical given the variability in weight and development among children. For instance, a medication dose for a 5-year-old who weighs 20 kg would be significantly different from that of a 2-year-old who weighs 10 kg, even if they were prescribed the same drug.

Body surface area (BSA) is another method used, particularly in chemotherapy and certain other treatments where the metabolic rate of tissue is a significant factor. The BSA method provides a more precise calculation, especially for drugs with a narrow therapeutic index. The formula commonly used is the Mosteller formula:

$$BSA(m^2) = \sqrt{\left(\frac{height(cm) \times weight(kg)}{3600}\right)}$$

This calculation helps ensure that the dosage is both safe and effective, minimizing the risk of toxicity or therapeutic failure.

Considerations for Developmental Stages

Children's bodies change rapidly as they grow, and their ability to metabolize medications evolves over time. Newborns and infants, for example, have immature liver and kidney functions, which affects how drugs are metabolized and excreted. This means that even medications commonly used in older children or adults might require adjustments in younger patients to avoid harmful accumulation.

As children age, their metabolic rates and organ functions mature, altering the way medications are processed. Therefore, a drug that is safe for a 10-year-old may require a different dosage for a toddler or an adolescent. Understanding these developmental differences is crucial when calculating dosages to ensure that the medication is appropriate for the child's age and stage of development.

Strategies for Safe Calculations and Administration

To safely calculate and administer medications to children, the following strategies should be employed:

1. **Use Weight-Based Calculations**: Always calculate doses based on the child's current weight, and update this information regularly to ensure accuracy.

2. **Double-Check Calculations**: Pediatric dosing often involves small volumes and precise measurements. Double-checking calculations, especially in critical medications, can prevent errors.

3. **Use Pediatric-Specific Tools**: Utilize pediatric dosing charts, online calculators, and apps that are specifically designed for pediatric calculations to streamline the process and reduce errors.

4. **Consult Guidelines**: Refer to up-to-date pediatric dosing guidelines from reputable sources, such as the American Academy of Pediatrics (AAP) or the World Health Organization (WHO), to ensure adherence to best practices.

5. **Involve Caregivers**: Educate parents or caregivers on the correct dosage and administration techniques, especially for at-home medications, to ensure continuity and safety.

Pediatric dosage calculations require careful consideration of the child's weight, surface area, and developmental stage. By applying these principles and strategies, nurses can ensure that children receive the correct dosages, maximizing therapeutic benefits while minimizing risks. These tailored approaches are essential for providing safe and effective care to our youngest patients.

4.2 Geriatric Dosages

Calculating dosages for elderly patients involves a distinct set of challenges due to the physiological changes that accompany aging. These changes affect how drugs are absorbed, distributed, metabolized, and excreted, making accurate dosage calculations essential to avoid adverse effects and ensure therapeutic efficacy.

Physiological Changes in Aging

As patients age, several physiological changes can significantly impact drug pharmacokinetics:

1. **Absorption**: Aging often leads to decreased gastric acid production and slower gastrointestinal motility, which can affect the rate and extent of drug absorption. For instance, medications that require an acidic environment for absorption, such as certain antifungals, may be less effective in elderly patients.

2. **Distribution**: Elderly patients generally have an increased body fat percentage and decreased lean body mass and total body water. These changes can alter the volume of distribution for many drugs, particularly those that are lipophilic (fat-soluble). For example, fat-soluble drugs like diazepam may have prolonged effects due to increased storage in adipose tissue.

3. **Metabolism**: Liver function typically declines with age, leading to reduced metabolic clearance of drugs. This can prolong the half-life of medications, increasing the risk of accumulation and toxicity, especially for drugs metabolized by the liver, such as warfarin and benzodiazepines.

4. **Excretion**: Kidney function also declines with age, which can result in decreased renal clearance of drugs. Medications that are primarily excreted by the kidneys, like digoxin and certain antibiotics, may require dose adjustments to prevent toxicity.

Polypharmacy and Drug Interactions

Polypharmacy, the use of multiple medications by a single patient, is common among the elderly and poses significant risks for drug interactions and adverse effects. Each additional medication increases the complexity of managing dosages and the potential for harmful interactions. For example, combining antihypertensive drugs with diuretics may lead to significant electrolyte imbalances or hypotension.

Careful review of all medications, including over-the-counter drugs and supplements, is crucial in geriatric patients. Regular medication reconciliation should be conducted to identify and eliminate unnecessary drugs, reduce the risk of interactions, and simplify the regimen where possible.

Practical Tips for Adjusting Dosages

1. **Start Low, Go Slow**: Initiate therapy at the lowest possible dose and titrate slowly, monitoring the patient's response to minimize the risk of adverse effects. This approach is particularly important for drugs with a narrow therapeutic index.

2. **Regular Monitoring**: Frequent monitoring of drug levels, renal function, and liver enzymes is essential to adjust dosages appropriately and avoid toxicity. For example, elderly patients on anticoagulants like warfarin should have their INR levels checked regularly to ensure safe and effective dosing.

3. **Use Geriatric Dosing Guidelines**: Refer to geriatric dosing guidelines that account for age-related changes in drug metabolism and excretion. These guidelines provide recommendations for dose adjustments based on the patient's renal and hepatic function.

4. **Simplify the Medication Regimen**: Whenever possible, simplify the medication regimen to improve adherence and reduce the risk of errors. This might involve using combination drugs, reducing the number of doses per day, or eliminating unnecessary medications.

Dosage calculations in elderly patients require a nuanced approach that accounts for the physiological changes of aging, the risks of polypharmacy, and the need for careful monitoring. By adjusting dosages thoughtfully and employing strategies to mitigate risks, healthcare providers can maximize the efficacy of medications while minimizing potential side effects, ultimately improving outcomes for geriatric patients.

4.3 Emergency Situations

In emergency medicine, the stakes are high, and the pace is relentless. Nurses often face situations where rapid medication administration is critical, and there is little room for error. In these high-pressure environments, accurate dosage calculations become a matter of life and death, requiring quick thinking and precise execution.

The Fast-Paced Environment

Emergency situations demand immediate action. Whether it's a cardiac arrest, anaphylactic shock, or acute respiratory distress, decisions must be made in seconds. The urgency of these scenarios leaves little time for detailed calculations or second-guessing, making the ability to quickly and accurately determine dosages essential.

For example, during a code blue, when a patient experiences cardiac arrest, medications like epinephrine must be administered within seconds. The nurse must be able to calculate the correct dose based on the patient's weight and administer it immediately, all while coordinating with the rest of the medical team.

Use of Standard Doses and Pre-Calculated Charts

To facilitate rapid medication administration, emergency departments often rely on standard doses and pre-calculated charts. These tools streamline the process, reducing the cognitive load on healthcare providers during critical moments.

1. **Standard Doses**: Many emergency medications, such as epinephrine, atropine, and naloxone, have established standard doses based on patient weight or age. These standard doses allow for quick administration without the need for complex calculations. For example, in pediatric emergencies, the Broselow tape is a widely used tool that provides weight-based dosing guidelines for various emergency medications, ensuring accurate and rapid dosing.

2. **Pre-Calculated Charts**: Pre-calculated dosage charts are another valuable resource in emergencies. These charts provide ready-to-use dose information for common medications, based on typical patient weights and scenarios. By referencing these charts, nurses can quickly determine the appropriate dose and administer it without delay.

These tools are not only time-saving but also help reduce the risk of calculation errors in high-stress situations, ensuring that patients receive the correct medication at the right dose.

Stress Management Techniques

Maintaining accuracy under pressure is a critical skill in emergency medicine. The high-stakes nature of the work can lead to stress, which, if not managed properly, can impair cognitive function and lead to errors. Here are some strategies to help maintain focus and accuracy:

1. **Practice and Drills**: Regular participation in emergency simulations and drills can help nurses become more familiar with emergency protocols and dosage calculations. Repeated exposure to these scenarios builds muscle memory, allowing for faster and more accurate responses in real situations.

2. **Controlled Breathing**: In the heat of the moment, taking a brief second to engage in controlled breathing can help calm nerves and clear the mind. This technique can reduce stress levels, allowing for better concentration and decision-making.

3. **Team Communication**: Clear and concise communication with the healthcare team is essential. Verbalizing calculations, confirming doses with a colleague, and listening to feedback can all help ensure that the correct dosage is administered.

Emergency situations require rapid, accurate medication administration, often under extreme pressure. Utilizing standard doses, pre-calculated charts, and effective stress management techniques can help nurses maintain accuracy and deliver life-saving care in these critical moments. Preparing for these scenarios through practice and teamwork is key to managing the demands of emergency medicine effectively.

4.4 High-Risk Medications

High-risk medications are those that have a significant potential for causing serious harm if administered incorrectly. These drugs often have a narrow therapeutic index, meaning the difference between a therapeutic dose and a toxic dose is very small. Additionally, they may have a high potential for adverse effects or require precise dosing based on individual patient factors. Administering these medications requires meticulous attention to detail, rigorous double-checking, and vigilant monitoring to ensure patient safety.

What Makes a Medication High-Risk?

Several characteristics can classify a medication as high-risk:

1. **Narrow Therapeutic Index**: Medications like warfarin, digoxin, and insulin have a narrow margin between therapeutic and toxic levels. Small deviations in dosage can lead to ineffective treatment or severe toxicity.

2. **High Potential for Adverse Effects**: Drugs such as opioids, anticoagulants, and chemotherapy agents are known for their significant side effect profiles, making accurate dosing critical to minimize harm.

3. **Complex Dosing Requirements**: Some medications, like heparin or vancomycin, require dosing adjustments based on patient-specific factors like renal function, weight, or serum levels, adding complexity to their administration.

Strategies for Accurate Calculations and Administration

Given the risks associated with these medications, it is essential to employ strategies that enhance accuracy and safety:

1. **Double-Checking**: Always have a second healthcare professional independently verify dosage calculations for high-risk medications. This practice is especially important for drugs with narrow therapeutic windows, where even minor errors can have serious consequences. For example, before administering insulin or anticoagulants, have a colleague review the dosage calculation and preparation to ensure accuracy.

2. **Use of Calculation Aids**: Utilize technology aids, such as digital calculators, dosing apps, or electronic health record (EHR) systems with built-in safety checks, to confirm dosage calculations. These tools can help prevent errors by providing immediate feedback if a calculation appears outside the recommended range.

3. **Tailored Dosing**: Adjust doses based on individual patient characteristics, such as age, weight, renal and

hepatic function, and current medications. For example, when administering vancomycin, dose adjustments may be necessary based on renal function and serum trough levels, requiring careful calculation and monitoring.

Protocols for Handling and Documentation

Adhering to strict protocols when administering high-risk medications is vital for patient safety:

1. **Standardized Procedures**: Follow standardized procedures for the preparation and administration of high-risk medications. These protocols should include steps for verifying patient identity, dosage calculations, and administration routes.

2. **Documenting Administration**: Accurate documentation is crucial for tracking the administration of high-risk medications. Record the dosage, time of administration, route, and any observed patient responses in the patient's medical record. This documentation not only ensures continuity of care but also provides a legal record of the treatment provided.

3. **Monitoring Patient Responses**: After administering high-risk medications, closely monitor the patient for any signs of adverse effects or unexpected responses. For example, when administering anticoagulants like warfarin, monitor the patient's INR levels and watch for signs of bleeding. Promptly report any concerns to the prescribing physician.

Handling high-risk medications requires a thorough understanding of their unique challenges, including their narrow therapeutic index and potential for serious adverse effects. By employing careful calculation strategies, double-checking processes, and adhering to strict protocols, healthcare providers can minimize risks and ensure the safe administration of these critical medications. Accurate documentation and vigilant monitoring further enhance patient safety and contribute to positive outcomes.

Chapter 5: Building Confidence and Competence

Mastering dosage calculations is about more than just getting the numbers right; it's about developing the confidence to trust your calculations in real-world situations. Confidence in dosage calculations doesn't come from memorizing formulas but from understanding the principles and knowing that you can apply them accurately, even under pressure.

As you transition from classroom learning to clinical practice, the ability to move from theoretical knowledge to practical assurance becomes crucial. Every nurse must reach a point where they not only perform calculations correctly but do so with the certainty that those calculations are reliable and safe. This chapter focuses on building both competence and confidence, guiding you through the steps to solidify your skills and trust your judgment.

We'll explore how to develop intuitive reasoning, the importance of continuous learning, and the tools and strategies that can help reinforce your abilities. By the end of this chapter, you'll have a clear understanding of how to confidently apply your dosage calculation skills in any clinical setting, ensuring the highest standard of patient care.

5.1 Developing Intuition

Developing intuition for dosage calculations is a critical step in becoming a proficient nurse. Intuition in this context isn't about guessing—it's about honing a deep, almost instinctual understanding of calculations that comes from repeated practice and experience. This intuition allows nurses to perform calculations quickly and accurately, even in high-pressure situations.

Building Intuition Through Practice and Exposure

Intuition is built through repetitive practice and exposure to a wide variety of clinical scenarios. The more you engage with dosage calculations, the more familiar and automatic they become. Start with the basics, practicing calculations daily until they feel second nature. Over time, challenge yourself with increasingly complex scenarios, such as adjusting doses based on patient-specific factors like weight, age, or kidney function.

Using case studies, simulation exercises, and real-life scenarios can significantly enhance this process. These methods expose you to different patient needs and medication requirements, helping you recognize patterns and common pitfalls. The goal is to reach a point where you can quickly assess a situation and accurately calculate the correct dosage without needing to rely heavily on formulas or references.

The Role of Mentorship and Experiential Learning

Mentorship plays a vital role in developing intuitive skills. Experienced nurses can provide guidance, share practical tips, and offer feedback on your calculation methods. Working closely with a mentor allows you to learn from their experience, observing how they approach dosage calculations in various situations. This hands-on learning is invaluable, as it gives you the opportunity to apply theoretical knowledge in real-time under the supervision of someone who has mastered the skill.

Experiential learning—learning by doing—is another powerful tool. Engaging in clinical rotations, internships, or simulations where you actively participate in dosage calculations reinforces your learning. Each experience builds your confidence, helping you to develop a "feel" for what's right. This experiential knowledge accumulates, shaping your intuition and enabling you to make quick, accurate decisions in practice.

Enhancing Speed and Accuracy with Intuitive Reasoning

Intuitive reasoning enhances both speed and accuracy in clinical settings. For example, when dealing with an emergency, there's no time to slowly work through a complex formula. An intuitive understanding allows you to make swift, accurate calculations based on your previous experiences and practice. If you've consistently calculated dosages for similar patients or medications, your brain starts recognizing the patterns, allowing you to perform calculations almost automatically.

Consider a nurse in an emergency room who, through experience and practice, can rapidly calculate and administer the correct dose of epinephrine during a cardiac arrest. Their intuition, built over time, ensures the patient receives the medication quickly and safely—potentially saving their life.

Developing intuition for dosage calculations is essential for any nurse aiming to provide high-quality care. Through repetitive practice, varied exposure, mentorship, and experiential learning, you can build the intuitive reasoning that enhances both speed and accuracy in clinical settings. This intuition is what will set you apart as a confident and competent nurse, capable of making critical decisions with assurance.

5.2 Continuous Learning and Improvement

Mastery in dosage calculations is not a one-time achievement; it requires continuous learning and adaptation. The healthcare field is constantly evolving, with new medications, technologies, and calculation methods emerging regularly. As a nurse, staying updated is crucial for maintaining your competence and ensuring patient safety.

Importance of Staying Updated

Medications are frequently updated or replaced, and new drugs with unique dosage requirements are introduced. Additionally, advancements in technology bring new tools and apps designed to aid in dosage calculations, making it essential to stay informed about the latest developments. Keeping up with these changes ensures that your skills remain relevant and that you can confidently handle any new challenges in clinical practice.

For example, understanding how to use the latest drug calculation apps or being aware of updates to dosing guidelines for a commonly used medication like insulin can significantly improve your efficiency and accuracy. Staying current also reduces the risk of errors that could arise from outdated knowledge or practices.

Strategies for Self-Assessment and Improvement

Continuous improvement begins with self-assessment. Regularly evaluate your dosage calculation skills to identify any areas where you might need further practice or learning. Start by reflecting on recent clinical experiences—were there any calculations you found challenging? Did you encounter any new medications that required additional research? Use these reflections to guide your learning.

Another effective strategy is to engage in peer reviews. Discuss your calculations with colleagues or mentors and ask for feedback. This collaborative approach not only helps you identify weaknesses but also exposes you to different perspectives and techniques that you might not have considered.

Keep a log of the calculations you perform regularly, noting any mistakes or uncertainties. Review this log periodically to track your progress and pinpoint recurring challenges. This habit allows you to focus your efforts on specific areas, ensuring continuous improvement.

Resources for Continuous Education

To maintain and enhance your skills, take advantage of the many resources available for continuous education.

1. **Workshops and Seminars**: Attend workshops and seminars that focus on dosage calculations or pharmacology. These events often provide hands-on learning experiences and the opportunity to interact with experts in the field.

2. **Online Courses**: Numerous online platforms offer courses in dosage calculations, often updated to include the latest practices and technologies. Websites like Coursera, Khan Academy, and specialized nursing education platforms offer flexible learning opportunities that can fit around your schedule.

3. **Professional Journals**: Regularly read professional journals like the *American Journal of Nursing* or *Nurse Educator*. These publications often feature articles on new medications, updated dosage guidelines, and the latest research in pharmacology, helping you stay informed and prepared.

4. **Simulation Software**: Utilize simulation software that replicates real-life scenarios, allowing you to practice dosage calculations in a controlled, risk-free environment. These tools can be particularly useful for reinforcing new skills or addressing specific challenges identified in self-assessments.

Continuous learning and improvement are essential for maintaining competence in dosage calculations. By staying updated with new developments, regularly assessing your skills, and utilizing educational resources, you can ensure that you provide safe, effective, and up-to-date care throughout your nursing career. This commitment to ongoing education not only enhances your professional growth but also significantly contributes to patient safety and positive outcomes.

5.3 Simulation and Practice Tools

Simulation and practice tools are invaluable resources for mastering dosage calculations. These tools offer hands-on, practical experiences that bridge the gap between theoretical knowledge and clinical application, allowing you to build confidence and competence in a controlled environment.

Types of Simulation Tools

There are various simulation tools available to help nursing students refine their dosage calculation skills:

1. **Software Programs**: Programs like *DoseCalc* and *PharmaSim* provide realistic scenarios where you can practice calculating doses based on patient-specific information. These programs often include instant feedback, helping you learn from mistakes in real-time.

2. **Interactive Online Platforms**: Platforms such as *NurseMath* and *NursingCalculations* offer a range of practice problems, quizzes, and interactive modules tailored to different levels of difficulty. These platforms allow you to progressively challenge yourself as your skills improve.

3. **Virtual Reality (VR) Simulations**: Some institutions offer VR simulations that immerse you in a virtual clinical environment. This advanced technology allows you to practice dosage calculations as part of a broader patient care scenario, enhancing both your technical skills and situational awareness.

Benefits of Using Simulation Tools

Simulation tools provide several key benefits:

- **Immediate Feedback**: Receiving instant feedback helps reinforce correct methods and corrects errors before they become ingrained habits.

- **Repetition and Consistency**: You can repeat scenarios as many times as needed, ensuring that you develop a consistent, reliable approach to dosage calculations.

- **Safe Environment**: Simulations allow you to make mistakes and learn from them without risking patient safety, which is critical during the learning process.

Real-Life Impact

Many nursing students report significant improvements in both competence and confidence after using simulation tools. For example, a student who struggled with weight-based dosing scenarios found that after several weeks of using an interactive platform, their accuracy improved dramatically, leading to better performance in clinical settings. These tools not only enhance your technical skills but also prepare you mentally for the fast-paced environment of real-world healthcare.

5.4 Preparing for Exams

Preparing for exams that test your dosage calculation skills requires focused study habits and effective revision techniques. Success in these exams not only reflects your knowledge but also your ability to apply it under pressure.

Effective Study Habits

1. **Regular Practice**: Consistent practice is key. Dedicate time each day to solving dosage problems, gradually increasing the difficulty level as you progress. This helps reinforce your understanding and builds speed.

2. **Use Flashcards**: Create flashcards for common dosage formulas, conversion factors, and key concepts. Flashcards are a great way to reinforce memory through repetition and can be easily used during short study breaks.

3. **Group Study**: Studying with peers allows you to discuss challenging problems and learn from each other's

perspectives. Group study sessions can also simulate the collaborative nature of clinical environments.

Approaching Exam Questions

When tackling exam questions, it's important to:

- **Read Carefully**: Misreading questions is a common pitfall. Pay close attention to details like units, patient weight, and the medication's concentration.

- **Double-Check Calculations**: Always review your calculations for errors. Simple mistakes in addition or unit conversion can lead to incorrect answers.

- **Prioritize Time**: Start with questions you find easier to build confidence, then move on to more challenging ones. This helps ensure you complete the exam efficiently.

Importance of Practice Exams

Practice exams are an excellent way to prepare for the real thing. They simulate the pressure of a timed test, helping you get comfortable with the exam format and time constraints. By taking practice exams regularly, you can identify areas where you need further study and refine your test-taking strategies.

Simulation tools and effective exam preparation strategies are critical to mastering dosage calculations. Through consistent practice, focused study, and the use of advanced learning tools, you can develop the competence and confidence needed to excel in exams and, ultimately, in your nursing career.

Conclusion

Mastering dosage calculations is a critical skill for any nursing student, and throughout this book, you've journeyed from foundational concepts to advanced applications in clinical settings. We've explored how to confidently calculate doses without relying on complex formulas, allowing you to approach every patient with the assurance that your calculations are both accurate and safe. From understanding the nuances of pediatric and geriatric dosing to handling emergencies and high-risk medications, you now have the tools and techniques to excel in your nursing practice.

The formula-free approach we've discussed not only simplifies the calculation process but also fosters a deeper understanding of how to apply these skills intuitively. This method enhances your ability to respond quickly and accurately in any situation, a crucial aspect of delivering high-quality patient care.

As you move forward, remember that continuous practice is key to maintaining and improving these skills. Approach every calculation with the confidence that you've developed through your hard work and dedication. The knowledge you've gained here is just the beginning—use it as a foundation for lifelong learning and professional growth.

For those seeking to expand their knowledge further, consider exploring additional resources such as professional workshops, online courses, and membership in nursing organizations. Stay engaged with the latest developments in medication administration, and never stop refining your skills.

Your commitment to mastering dosage calculations is a testament to your dedication to patient safety and excellence in nursing. Keep pushing forward, and let the confidence you've built through this book guide you in your future endeavors.

www.ingramcontent.com/pod-product-compliance
Lightning Source LLC
Chambersburg PA
CBHW071123240526

45465CB00023B/786